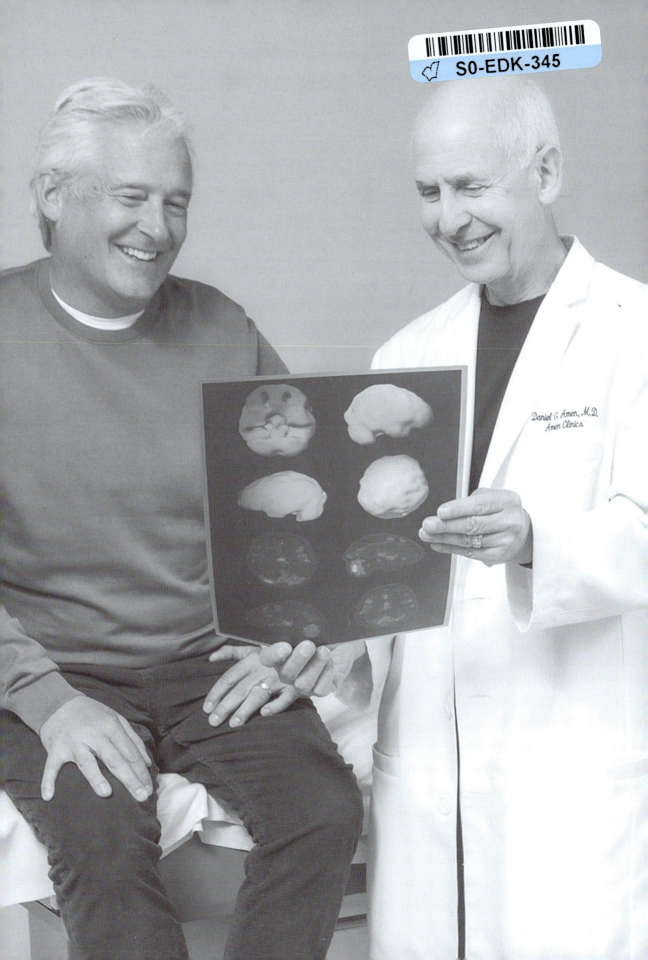

CONTENTS

INTRODUCTION

INTRODUCTION

How to Use This Memory Makeover Workbook

Congratulations on taking this vital step to tackle memory problems—or the possibility of them down the road—before it is too late! Memory is one of the most important functions of the brain, and problems with it are becoming increasingly common, even among teenagers and young adults. Did you know that 80% of people who have had COVID-19 later complain of memory and focus issues? Forgetfulness gets much worse with age, but memory loss is not normal. And it is not inevitable.

This step-by-step workbook is designed to help you on the path to a healthier brain, a better memory, and a happier, more fulfilling life. You are not stuck with the brain you have, you can make it better, but you have to work to change your brain every day.

Identifying and treating all the risk factors for memory problems as soon as possible is the best way to prevent and even reverse them. BRIGHT MINDS is the mnemonic (memory device) used at Amen Clinics that sums up the 11 major risk factors that can hurt your brain and diminish your memory.

The BRIGHT MINDS risk factors you will learn more about in this workbook and that are key to addressing memory issue are:

B — Blood Flow
R — Retirement/Aging
I — Inflammation
G — Genetics
H — Head Trauma
T — Toxins

M — Mental Health
I — Immunity/Infections
N — Neurohormone Issues
D — Diabesity
S — Sleep Issues

The good news is that almost all these risk factors are either preventable or treatable, and even the ones that aren't, such as having a family history of dementia (genetics), can be improved with the right strategies. This workbook provides you with all the strategies you need to address your personal risks.

Which Brain Do You Want?

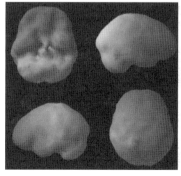

Healthy
Full, even, symmetrical blood flow

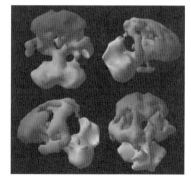

Classic Alzheimer's Disease
Decreases in parietal/temporal lobes

STEP 1
ASSESS THE CURRENT HEALTH OF YOUR BRAIN AND MEMORY

How well do you think your brain is working? What about your memory? The results of the following questionnaires will help you know where to devote your health-improvement efforts. You will start by assessing how your brain, memory, and health are right now. The following assessment tools are the same ones we use at Amen Clinics with all our patients who come in with memory problems. Take the time to fill them out now, and then do them again in 30 days to see the progress you have made.

ASSESSMENT 1.
Do You Have Any Early Warning Signs of Memory Problems?

Problems in the brain usually begin years before you show any symptoms. That's why it is so important to recognize the early warning signs. This first self-assessment includes questions relating to the most critical of these signs. (Scoring follows the questions.)

Answer each question with a number from 0-4, ranging from Never (0) to Very Frequently (4).

0	1	2	3	4
Never	Rarely	Occassionally	Frequently	Very Frequently

PROBLEMS WITH YOUR MEMORY—DO YOU:

——— 1. Tend to be forgetful?
——— 2. Notice that your memory, although never good, has gotten worse?
——— 3. Misplace your keys or wallet?
——— 4. Wonder why you came into a room?
——— 5. Have trouble remembering names?
——— 6. Feel embarrassed about forgetting appointments?
——— 7. Read a book or an article, but don't remember much of it?
——— 8. Have trouble remembering things that happened recently?

PROBLEMS WITH YOUR MEMORY—DO YOU:

_____ 9. Struggle with brain fog?
_____ 10. Have trouble remembering to take medications or supplements?
_____ 11. Rely more and more on memory aids or reminders on your phone?
_____ 12. Know something one day but forget it the next?
_____ 13. Forget what you're going to say right in the middle of saying it?
_____ 14. Have trouble following directions that have more than one or two steps?
_____ 15. Worry that your memory is worse than it was 10 years ago?
_____ 16. Lose track of the conversation?
_____ 17. Find things in unusual places, like your keys in the refrigerator?
_____ 18. Get mad at others, thinking they took your things, only to find out later you misplaced them?

PLANNING AND PROBLEM-SOLVING ISSUES—DO YOU:

_____ 19. Have trouble making plans and sticking to them?
_____ 20. Find It harder to follow a recipe or directions on putting something together?
_____ 21. Find it hard to focus on more complex tasks, especially those that involve math? For example, are you struggling with managing your bills or balancing your checkbook?

MIX-UPS WITH TIMES AND PLACES—DO YOU:

_____ 22. Have trouble driving to locations that were once familiar to you?
_____ 23. Get easily confused or out of sorts?
_____ 24. Get more easily lost or have to rely on a GPS more than before?

ISSUES WITH WORDS—DO YOU:

_____ 25. Struggle to find the right word?
_____ 26. Call things by the wrong name?
_____ 27. Avoid joining conversations with people?
_____ 28. Have trouble following along in conversations?
_____ 29. Keep repeating yourself?

JUDGMENT ISSUES—DO YOU:

_____ 30. Struggle with making more bad decisions?
_____ 31. Make mistakes with your finances?

WITHDRAWING SOCIALLY—DO YOU:

_____ 32. Feel more isolated from friends?
_____ 33. Feel like cutting back at work because you just don't care as much?
_____ 34. Feel less interested in activities you usually find fun?
_____ 35. Take less care of your physical appearance?

SCORING:

Add up the number of questions to which you answered 3 (Frequently) or 4 (Very Frequently), then check the total against the key.

KEY:

0	1-2	3-5	6 or higher
Low risk of significant memory issues	Mild risk of having significant memory issues	Moderate risk of having significant memory issues	High risk of having significant memory issues

ASSESSMENT 2.

How is Your Brain Functioning?

Cognitive testing can tell you how your brain is currently functioning compared to other people your age. Several cognitive tests are available online; the one we use at Amen Clinics is called BrainFit WebNeuro, which you can access for free through our BrainFitLife program at www.brainfitlife.com. The test takes a little more than 30 minutes to complete, measures an extensive number of cognitive and emotional functions, and produces an objective assessment of how your brain is working in 17 specific areas. Each area is scored on a scale of 1 to 10, and you'll get an overall brain health score too. Any individual scores that are below 5 should raise a red flag.

One of the great things about this kind of testing is that it gives you a baseline score and, through repeat testing, a way to determine whether your brain is getting better (or worse) over time.

Take this test (or another cognitive test) now and repeat it in 30 days to chart your progress.

MY COGNITIVE TESTS	MY SCORE NOW:	MY FOLLOW-UP SCORE:
MOTOR COORDINATION		
PROCESSING SPEED (HOW QUICKLY YOU PROCESS INFORMATION)		
SUSTAINED ATTENTION (MAINTAIN FOCUS)		
CONTROLLED ATTENTION (ABILITY TO STOP REACTIONS WHEN NEEDED)		
FLEXIBILITY (SHIFTING ATTENTION)		
INHIBITION (SELF-CONTROL)		
WORKING MEMORY (HOLD INFORMATION FOR SHORT PERIODS)		
RECALL MEMORY (REMEMBER INFORMATION)		
EXECUTIVE FUNCTION (PLAN AND ORGANIZE INFORMATION)		
IDENTIFY EMOTIONS (READING FACES)		
EMOTION BIAS (IMPACT OF EMOTIONS ON DECISION MAKING)		
STRESS LEVEL		
ANXIETY LEVEL		
DEPRESSED MOOD LEVEL		
POSITIVITY-NEGATIVITY BIAS (TENDENCY TO NOTICE POSITIVE OR NEGATIVE EMOTIONS)		
RESILIENCE (COPING DURING DIFFICULT TIMES)		
SOCIAL CAPACITY (BUILDING AND KEEPING RELATIONSHIPS)		
OVERALL BRAIN HEALTH		

ASSESSMENT 3.

What Is Your Risk for Memory Problems?

More than 6.5 people in the U.S. have Alzheimer's disease—the most common type of dementia—and that number is expected to more than double by the year 2050. It is the sixth leading cause of death, and despite the hundreds of experimental drugs developed over the past two decades to treat it, there is still no cure.

Research has confirmed that the best way to prevent Alzheimer's and memory loss is to prevent all the conditions that put you at risk for it. Therefore, if you want to keep your brain healthy as you get older, it is critical to avoid the risk factors as much as possible.

According to the BRIGHT MINDS formula, here are the 11 risk factor categories. Each contributing factor has been given a numerical weighting that indicates how harmful it may be to your brain and memory. Check off the contributing risks you know apply to you. If there are ones you are not sure about, you may need to schedule an appointment with your doctor to have certain lab tests done. The number in the right column is the relative increase in risk for memory problems, accelerated aging, and Alzheimer's disease compared to people who don't have that risk factor. When you have finished this questionnaire, tally your score.

This is what the numbers mean:

1.3 = 30% increased risk
1.7 = 70% increased risk
2 = twice the risk
4 = quadruple the risk, and on up to 38 = 38 times the risk!

BLOOD FLOW RISK FACTORS

☐ History of a stroke	5
☐ History of cardiovascular disease, including coronary artery disease, heart attacks, heart failure, heart arrhythmias	2
☐ Prehypertension or hypertension in midlife	2
☐ Low blood pressure in later life	1.3
☐ Erectile dysfunction	
• All Ages	1.7
• Age 50 to 64	6.1
• Over age 65	27.2
☐ Limited exercise (under 2 times a week)	2

RETIREMENT/AGING RISK FACTORS

☐ Age 65 to 84 ————————————————————→ 2

☐ Age 85 and older ————————————————————→ 38

☐ Watching too much television (more than 2 hours a day) ——————→ 2

☐ A job that does not require new learning, or being retired
without new opportunities for learning ————————————→ 2

☐ Loneliness or social isolation ————————————————→ 2

INFLAMMATION RISK FACTORS

☐ Periodontal (gum) disease ————————————————————→ 2

☐ Presence of inflammation in the body, such as high
homocysteine or C-reactive protein ————————————→ 2

☐ Low omega-3 fatty acids (from Omega-3 Index test) ——————————→ 2

GENETICS RISK FACTORS

☐ One family member with Alzheimer's or dementia ————————————→ 3.5

☐ More than one family member with Alzheimer's or dementia ——————→ 7.5

☐ One apolipoprotein e4 (APOE4) gene (if known, based on genetic testing)——→ 2.5

☐ Two APOE4 genes (if known, based on genetic testing) ———————→ 10

HEAD TRAUMA RISK FACTORS

☐ A single head injury with loss of consciousness ————————————→ 2

☐ Several head injuries without a loss of consciousness ————————→ 2

☐ Loss of one's sense of smell ————————————————————→ 2

TOXIN RISK FACTORS

☐ Smoking cigarettes for 10 years or longer (currently or in past) ——————→ 2.3

☐ Alcohol dependence or drug dependence (currently or in past) ——————→ 4.4

☐ History of radiation for head and neck cancers ————————————→ 3

☐ History of chemotherapy

    • For breast cancer ————————————————————→ 1.5

    • For colorectal cancer, possibly other cancers ————————→ 1.25

☐ Chronic exposure to heavy metals, such as lead, cadmium, mercury, or aluminum ——→ 1.5

☐ Chronic mold exposure ————————————————————→ 1.5

☐ Kidney dysfunction ————————————————————→ 2

MENTAL HEALTH RISK FACTORS

- ☐ PTSD — 4
- ☐ Bipolar disorder — 2
- ☐ Schizophrenia — 2
- ☐ Depression — 3.5
- ☐ Chronic stress — 2
- ☐ Childhood trauma — 2

IMMUNITY/INFECTIONS RISK FACTORS

- ☐ Autoimmune issues, including
  - • Multiple sclerosis — 1.5
  - • Rheumatoid arthritis — 3
  - • Systemic lupus erythematosus — 2
  - • Crohn's disease — 1.5
  - • Severe psoriasis — 3
- ☐ Adult asthma — 1.3
- ☐ Chronic Lyme disease or other infectious process in brain/ body not fully treated — 2
- ☐ Cold sores or genital herpes — 2

NEUROHORMONE RISK FACTORS

- ☐ Low thyroid — 2
- ☐ Low estrogen (in females) — 2
- ☐ Low testosterone (males and females) — 2
- ☐ Hysterectomy without estrogen replacement — 2
- ☐ History of prostate cancer with testosterone-lowering treatment — 2

DIABESITY RISK FACTORS

- ☐ Pre-diabetes or diabetes — 3
- ☐ Being overweight or obese in middle age — 3
- ☐ Being underweight in older age — 2

SLEEP RISK FACTORS

- ☐ Chronic insomnia — 2.3
- ☐ Sleep apnea — 2

TOTAL YOUR SCORE:

Tally the number of risk factors you have checked off and then tally the numbers for the risk factors you checked (relative risk factors).

_____ Total number of risk factors (number of checked boxes) you have
_____ Relative risk factors (add the relevant numbers in the right-hand column)

HOW TO INTERPRET YOUR RELATIVE RISK FACTOR SCORE

0-6	7-14	14+
Low risk of significant memory issues	Mild risk of having significant memory issues	Moderate risk of having significant memory issues

*Annual screening should include lab tests, a repeat of cognitive testing, and a checkup with your healthcare provider.

ASSESSMENT 4.

What are Your Health "Stats"?

These numbers let you know how your body is functioning and are common yet important indicators of your overall health. In the chart that follows, enter the numbers that you know or can assess yourself; for those that you don't already know, ask your doctor to have your blood drawn or visit one of the Amen Clinics. Enter these numbers in the following chart when you receive your test results.

MY IMPORTANT HEALTH NUMBERS

Let's start with your Body Mass Index (BMI). Find your height in the left column, and then read across that row to find your weight. Your BMI is at the top of that column.

WEIGHT

lbs	4'8" 142cm	4'9" 149	4'10" 147	4'11" 150	5'0" 152	5'1" 155	5'2" 157	5'3" 160	5'4" 163	5'5" 165	5'6" 168	5'7" 170	5'8" 173	5'9" 175	5'10" 178	5'11" 180	6'0" 183	6'1" 185	6'2" 188	6'3" 191	6'4" 193	6'5" 196
260	58	56	54	53	51	49	48	46	45	43	42	41	40	38	37	36	35	34	33	32	32	31
255	57	55	53	51	50	48	47	45	44	42	41	40	39	38	37	36	35	34	33	32	31	30
250	56	54	52	50	49	47	46	44	43	42	40	39	38	37	36	35	34	33	32	31	30	30
245	55	53	51	49	48	46	45	43	42	41	40	38	37	36	35	34	33	32	31	31	30	29
240	54	52	50	48	47	45	44	43	41	40	39	38	36	35	34	33	33	32	31	30	29	28
235	53	51	49	47	46	44	43	42	40	39	38	37	36	35	34	33	32	31	30	29	29	28
230	52	50	48	46	45	43	42	41	39	38	37	36	35	34	33	32	31	30	30	29	28	27
225	50	49	47	45	44	43	41	40	39	37	36	35	34	33	32	31	31	30	29	28	27	27
220	49	48	46	44	43	42	40	39	38	37	36	34	33	32	32	31	30	29	28	27	27	26
215	48	47	45	43	42	41	39	38	37	36	35	34	33	32	31	30	29	28	28	27	26	25
210	47	45	44	42	41	40	38	37	36	35	34	33	32	31	30	29	28	28	27	26	26	25
205	46	44	43	41	40	39	37	36	35	34	33	32	31	30	29	29	28	27	26	26	25	24
200	45	43	42	40	39	38	37	35	34	33	32	31	30	30	29	28	27	26	26	25	24	24
195	44	42	41	39	38	37	36	35	33	32	31	31	30	29	28	27	26	26	25	24	24	23
190	43	41	40	38	37	36	35	34	33	32	31	30	29	28	27	26	26	25	24	24	23	23
185	41	40	39	37	36	35	34	33	32	31	30	29	28	27	27	26	25	24	24	23	23	22
180	40	39	38	36	35	34	33	32	31	30	29	28	27	27	26	25	24	24	23	22	22	21
175	39	38	37	35	34	33	32	31	30	29	28	27	27	26	25	24	24	23	22	22	21	21
170	38	37	36	34	33	32	31	30	29	28	27	27	26	25	24	24	23	22	22	21	21	20
165	37	36	34	33	32	31	30	29	28	27	27	26	25	24	24	23	22	22	21	21	20	20
160	36	35	33	32	31	30	29	28	27	27	26	25	24	24	23	22	22	21	21	20	19	19
155	35	34	32	31	30	29	28	27	27	26	25	24	24	23	22	22	21	20	20	19	19	18
150	34	32	31	30	29	28	27	27	26	25	24	23	23	22	22	21	20	20	19	19	18	18
145	33	31	30	29	28	27	27	26	25	24	23	23	22	21	21	20	20	19	19	18	18	17
140	31	30	29	28	27	26	26	25	24	23	23	22	21	21	20	20	19	18	18	17	17	17
135	30	29	28	27	26	26	25	24	23	22	22	21	21	20	19	19	18	18	17	17	16	16
130	29	28	27	26	25	25	24	23	22	22	21	20	20	19	19	18	18	17	17	16	16	15
125	28	27	26	25	24	24	23	22	21	21	20	20	19	18	18	17	17	16	16	16	15	15
120	27	26	25	24	23	23	22	21	21	20	19	19	18	18	17	17	16	16	15	15	15	14
115	26	25	24	23	22	22	21	20	20	19	19	18	17	17	16	16	16	15	15	14	14	14
110	25	24	23	22	21	21	20	19	19	18	18	17	17	16	16	15	15	15	14	14	13	13
105	24	23	22	21	21	20	19	19	18	17	17	16	16	16	15	15	14	14	13	13	13	12
100	22	22	21	20	20	19	18	18	17	17	16	16	15	15	14	14	14	13	13	12	12	12
95	21	21	20	19	19	18	17	17	16	16	15	15	14	14	14	13	13	13	12	12	12	11
90	20	19	19	18	18	17	16	16	15	15	15	14	14	13	13	13	12	12	11	11	11	11
85	19	18	18	17	17	16	16	15	15	14	14	13	13	13	12	12	12	11	11	11	10	10
80	18	17	17	16	16	15	15	14	14	13	13	13	12	12	11	11	11	11	10	10	10	9

My Body Mass Index Number: _____

BODY MASS INDEX (BMI)

Underweight: <18.5
Healthy weight: 18.5-24.9
Overweight: 25-30
Obese: greater than 30
Morbid obesity: 40 or higher

WAIST TO HEIGHT RATIO (WHtR)

Use a tape measure to measure at your belly button. For a healthy WHtR, your waist size should be half your height—or less—in inches

HEALTHY RATIO: Less than or equal to 0.5.

My WHtR Number: _____

BLOOD PRESSURE

OPTIMAL:

Systolic (top number): 90-120
Diastolic (bottom number): 60-80

My Blood Pressure Numbers: ___/___

LIPID PANEL (CHOLESTEROL)

Total cholesterol:

Normal: 160-200 mg/dL (below 160 has been associated with depression)

Optimal: 160-200 mg/dL

HDL: greater than or equal to 60 mg/dL
LDL: less than 100 mg/dL
Triglycerides: Less than 150 mg/dL

My Cholesterol Numbers:

Total____
HDL____
LDL____
Triglycerides____

HEMOGLOBIN A1C (HBA1C):

Normal: 4.0 – 5.6%
Prediabetes: 5.7 – 6.4%
Diabetes: Greater than 6.4%

My HbA1c Number: _____

My General Metabolic Numbers	GENERAL METABOLIC PANEL

My General Metabolic Numbers

Liver Function:

ALT (SGPT) _____
AST (SGOT) _____
Bilirubin_____
Zinc _____

Kidney Function:

BUN_____
Creatinine _____

GENERAL METABOLIC PANEL
(KIDNEY AND LIVER FUNCTION):

LIVER FUNCTION

ALT (SGPT): Normal range: 7 to 56 units per liter (U/L)

AST (SGOT): Normal range: 5 to 40 U/L

Bilirubin: Normal range: 0.2 to1.2 mg/dL

Zinc: Normal range: 60 to 110 mcg/dL (low zinc will limit detoxification in the liver)

KIDNEY FUNCTION

BUN: Normal range: 7 to 20 mg/dL

Creatinine: Normal range: 0.5 to 1.2 mg/dL

My Fasting Blood Sugar Number: _____

FASTING BLOOD SUGAR:

Normal: 70-105 mg/dL
Optimal: 70-85 mg/dL
Pre-diabetes: 105-125 mg/dL
Diabetes: 126 mg/dL or higher

My Homocysteine Number: _____

HOMOCYSTEINE:
Healthy level: less than 10 mmol/L

My CRP Number: _____

C-REACTIVE PROTEIN: (CRP)
Healthy range: 0.0 - 1.0 mg/dL

My Ferritin Number: _____

FERRITIN:
Ideal levels: 40–80 ng/mL

My Thyroid Numbers: TSH: _____ Free T3: _____ Free T4: _____	**THYROID:** **TSH (thyroid-stimulating hormone):** 0.4–3.0mIU/L **Free T3:** 100–200 ng/dL **Free T4:** 4.5–11.2 mcg/dL
My Free Serum Testosterone **Number:** _____ **My Total Serum Testosterone** **Number:** _____	**FREE & TOTAL SERUM TESTOSTERONE:** **Normal levels for women:** Free: 0.3-1.9 ng/dL Total: 8-60 ng/dL **Optimal levels for women:** Free: 0.8-1.9 ng/dL Total: 30-60 ng/dL **Normal levels for men:** Free: 9-30 ng/dL Total: 300-1100 ng/dL **Optimal levels for men:** Free: 15-30 ng/dL Total: 600-1100 ng/dL
My DHEA-S Number: _____	**DHEA-S:** **Normal:** 44–332 µg/dL
My Vitamin D Number: _____	**VITAMIN D:** **Low:** Below 30mg/dL **Optimal:** 50-100mg/dL

ASSESSMENT 5.

Did You Have Any Adverse Childhood Experiences (ACEs)?

If your childhood was marked by abuse, neglect, or other traumatic experiences, it can have a lasting negative impact on your health. The toxic stress that ACEs can cause may increase the risk for developing 7 of the top 10 leading causes of death, such as cancer, depression, and addiction—all of which can lead to memory problems later on.

My Adverse Childhood Experiences (ACEs)

To determine if and how many ACEs you had, put a checkmark next to any item in the questionnaire below that applies to you. Then add up the checkmarks to get your ACE score.

_____ 1. Before your 18th birthday, did a parent or other adult in the household often or very often: swear at you, insult you, put you down, or humiliate you? *OR* act in a way that made you afraid that you might be physically hurt?

_____ 2. Before your 18th birthday, did a parent or other adult in the household often or very often: push, grab, slap, or throw something at you? *OR* ever hit you so hard that you had marks or were injured?

_____ 3. Before your 18th birthday, did an adult or person at least five years older than you ever: touch or fondle you or have you touch their body in a sexual way? *OR* attempt to or have oral, anal, or vaginal intercourse with you?

_____ 4. Before your 18th birthday, did you often or very often feel that: no one in your family loved you or thought you were important or special? *OR* your family didn't look out for each other, feel close to each other, or support each other?

_____ 5. Before your 18th birthday, did you often or very often feel that: you didn't have enough to eat, had to wear dirty clothes, and had no one to protect you? *OR* your parents were too drunk or high to take care of you or take you to the doctor if you needed it?

_____ 6. Before your 18th birthday, was a biological parent ever lost to you through divorce, abandonment, or other reason?

_____ 7. Before your 18th birthday, was your mother or stepmother: often or very often pushed, grabbed, slapped, or had something thrown at her? *OR* sometimes, often, or very often kicked, bitten, hit with a fist, or hit with something hard? *OR* ever repeatedly hit for at least a few minutes or threatened with a gun or knife?

_____ 8. Before your 18th birthday, did you live with anyone who was a problem drinker or alcoholic, or who used street drugs?

_____ 9. Before your 18th birthday, was a household member depressed or mentally ill, or did a household member attempt suicide?

_____ 10. Before your 18th birthday, did a household member go to prison?

ACE SCORING

Add up the number of items you checked and enter it here _____. This is your ACE score.

SUMMARY OF SELF-ASSESSMENT TASKS

1. Note any signs of memory loss that you are experiencing.

2. Take an online cognitive test to see how your brain is functioning compared to others your age.

3. Find out what your personal BRIGHT MINDS risk factors and relative risks are.

4. Know your important health numbers and record them.

5. Know your ACEs score.

In Step 2, read through all 11 BRIGHT MINDS risk factors and check the boxes and make note of any risk factors that apply to you.

RISK FACTOR: BLOOD FLOW

Blood flow throughout your body brings oxygen and other nutrients to all your cells and carries away waste products. Surprisingly, the blood vessels that feed our brain cells age faster than the brain cells do, so keeping your brain healthy means taking care of your blood vessels. Low blood flow is the #1 brain imaging predictor of Alzheimer's disease.

YOUR PERSONAL RISK CHECKLIST:

Which Bloodflow Risk Factors Do You Have?

If you don't know whether you have any of the following risk factors, schedule a checkup with your healthcare provider who will take your blood pressure, listen to your heart, and order laboratory tests to assess the health of your blood vessels. You can always fill in this checklist when you have the results of your checkup and tests.

CARDIOVASCULAR DISEASE

- ☐ Atherosclerosis (hardening of the arteries)
- ☐ Atrial fibrillation
- ☐ Heart attack
- ☐ High LDL or total cholesterol
- ☐ Hypertension or prehypertension
  - Hypertensive: 140/90 mm/Hg or higher
  - Prehypertensive: 125/85 – 139/89 mm/Hg

OTHER RISK FACTORS

- [ ] Having a stroke or transient ischemic attack (TIA)

- [ ] Exercising less than twice a week and/or having a slow walking speed. Ultimately, one of the most important reasons to exercise is that it keeps your blood vessels open and healthy.

- [ ] Episode(s) of a loss of oxygen to the brain, such as during sleep apnea, a near drowning, or a heart attack when the heart stops beating

- [ ] Erectile dysfunction

KEY BLOOD FLOW TESTS

While it is important to know all your health numbers, the following ones are key to assessing the status of your circulatory system. Be sure to have these tests done now.

- [ ] Blood pressure: Both high (130/80 or higher) and low blood pressure (less than 90/60) are a problem

- [ ] CBC (complete blood count)

- [ ] Lipid panel: Cholesterol levels that are too high or too low are bad for the brain

RISK FACTOR: RETIREMENT/AGING

Advancing age is the single most important risk for memory loss and Alzheimer's disease. Did you know that 50% of people 85 and older will be diagnosed with Alzheimer's? This means if you're blessed to live to 85 or beyond, you have a 1 in 2 chance of losing your mind. Although true, it is not inevitable that your mental faculties have to decline with age. Keeping mentally fit means addressing the biological and emotional/psychological issues that arise as you get older.

YOUR PERSONAL RISK CHECKLIST:

Which Retirement/Aging Risk Factors Do You Have?

If you are unsure whether you have any of the following risk factors, schedule a checkup with your healthcare provider who can order laboratory tests for iron and other health measures related to aging. You can always fill in this checklist when you have the results of your checkup and tests.

- [ ] Age: I am ___ years old
- [ ] Retirement/lack of new learning
- [ ] Shortened telomeres (casings at the ends of chromosomes—determined by lab testing)
- [ ] Social isolation
- [ ] Too much (or too little) iron

KEY RETIREMENT/AGING TESTS

While it is important to know all your health numbers, the ones here are key to assessing how well you are aging. Be sure to have these tests done now.

- [ ] C-reactive protein (CRP): a measure of inflammation

- [ ] DHEA: Higher levels of this neurohormone, as well as testosterone, are associated with longevity

- [ ] Fasting blood sugar: This blood test, along with Hemoglobin A1c, screens for prediabetes and diabetes

- [ ] Ferritin (iron levels)

- [ ] Hemoglobin A1C (HbA1C)

- [ ] Testosterone

- [ ] Telomere length: Testing for CRP and HbA1C (see above) may be substituted for this test

---

Quick Memory Tip:

When you think or tell people you're too set in your ways, or too old or too tired to make changes, it can become self-fulfilling. So pay attention to your thoughts and words!

RISK FACTOR: INFLAMMATION

In Latin, inflammare means "to set on fire." It is the root of the word inflammation and is an accurate description of what chronic inflammation does inside your body. It is like a constant fire that harms your organs and blood vessels—and can destroy your brain.

YOUR PERSONAL RISK CHECKLIST:

Which Inflammation Risk Factors Do You Have?

While inflammation is your body's natural (and necessary) reaction to infection and injury, it's important to know what else can trigger inflammation and the conditions under which it can become chronic and harmful. Cigarette smoking, high blood sugar levels, exposure to environmental toxins, and gum disease are a few of the culprits.

The following are two major memory-harming sources of chronic inflammation:

☐ Leaky gut (when the lining of the gastrointestinal tract becomes permeable)

☐ Low omega-3 fatty acids (especially the fatty acids known as EPA and DHA)

KEY TESTS FOR INFLAMMATION

While it is important to know all your health numbers, the ones here are key to assessing whether or not inflammation is an issue for you. Be sure to have these blood tests done now.

☐ C-reactive protein (CRP)

☐ Folate

☐ Homocysteine

☐ Interleukin 6 (IL-6)

☐ Omega-3 Index: a measure of omega-3 fatty acids EPA and DHA in red blood cells, which reflects brain levels of these fats

☐ Vitamin B12

Quick Memory Tip:

Having a healthy gut is critical because good gut bacteria help protect you from illnesses, such as E. coli, and supports your mental health too!

RISK FACTOR: GENETICS

Having a family history of Alzheimer's disease or other forms of dementia increase your risk for memory problems. However, a genetic vulnerability is not a death sentence. It should be a wake-up call.

YOUR PERSONAL RISK CHECKLIST:

Which Genetic Risk Factors Do You Have?

In families that have severe memory problems, Alzheimer's disease, or another type of dementia, members are more at risk for memory troubles. The same is true for people who have one or two copies of the APOE4 gene or several other genes. It is therefore critical to know if any of your extended family members have problems with their memory and take steps to protect yours.

☐ A family history of memory problems, Alzheimer's, or another type of dementia

☐ One or two copies of the APOE4 gene

☐ Presenilin 1 or 2 genes

KEY GENETIC TESTS

☐ Apolipoprotein E (APOE) gene status

☐ Additional genetic testing for other genes like presenilin genes 1 and 2 if members of your family have early-onset memory problems; ask your doctor about this.

RISK FACTOR: HEAD TRAUMA

Numerous studies have shown that a head injury or multiple head injuries—including mild ones that don't cause you to black out or that aren't diagnosed as a concussion—are linked to a higher risk of memory problems. Those that occur early in life (before age 25) more than double the risk; those that happen later (after age 55) almost quadruple the risk.

YOUR PERSONAL RISK CHECKLIST:

Which Head Trauma Risk Factors Do You Have?

Brain tissue is soft, similar to the texture of custard, and the bony skull that protects the brain has sharp ridges on the inside. Therefore, anything that causes your brain to hit up against the inside of your skull can cause trauma—bruising, bleeding, lack of oxygen, damaged brain cells, and more. Here are a few of the things that can lead to this kind of head trauma:

- ☐ A fall (down steps, off a ladder, out of bed, in the bath or shower, out of a tree, etc.)
- ☐ A motor vehicle collision with a car, motorcycle, truck, bicycle, or ATV
- ☐ A pedestrian-vehicle collision
- ☐ Combat injuries, including being exposed to explosive blasts
- ☐ Sport injuries and concussions in football, soccer, hockey, boxing, baseball, basketball, cycling, etc.
- ☐ Violence (gunshot wounds, domestic violence, an assault, etc.)

KEY HEAD TRAUMA TESTS

- [ ] If you have had a head trauma and your memory isn't what you want it to be or if your thinking skills are impaired, consider getting a SPECT or qEEG scan

- [ ] Get your sense of smell evaluated if you are having trouble smelling peanut butter, lemon, strawberry, or natural gas scents

- [ ] Omega-3 Index: a measure of omega-3 fatty acids EPA and DHA in red blood cells, which reflects brain levels of these fats

- [ ] HbA1c and fasting blood sugar (high blood sugar levels can delay healing)

- [ ] Thyroid, DHEA-S, and testosterone levels (damage to the master hormone gland, the pituitary, can cause hormone deficiencies)

Quick Memory Tip:

Don't be afraid to tell your kids that you won't let them to play football. Let them know it can hurt their brain and lead to unhappiness and struggling in life. Give them options for other, less risky sports to play.

RISK FACTOR: TOXINS

Exposure to environmental toxins has been linked to health problems ranging from allergies and cancer to autoimmune and neurodegenerative diseases. That's because our bodies' systems to detoxify (through the gut, liver, kidneys, and skin), can become overwhelmed, damaging the brain, leading to serious illness, and increasing the risk of memory problems and dementia.

YOUR PERSONAL RISK CHECKLIST:

Which Toxins Have You Been Exposed To?

Toxins can be absorbed through your skin, ingested (when you eat or drink), or inhaled. You may have been exposed to a toxin once, on occasion, or continuously. Below is a partial list of what you may have been exposed to.

- [ ] Air pollution
- [ ] Artificial food dyes, preservatives, and sweeteners
- [ ] Asbestos
- [ ] BPA
- [ ] Carbon monoxide
- [ ] Chemotherapy
- [ ] Cigarette smoke
- [ ] Cleaning chemicals
- [ ] E-cigarette vapor
- [ ] Excessive alcohol
- [ ] Fire retardant fumes
- [ ] Fireplace fumes
- [ ] Gasoline fumes
- [ ] General anesthesia
- [ ] Health and beauty products, (such as lead in lip products and formaldehyde in nail polishes)

- [ ] Heavy metals (such as lead, mercury from dental fillings, or cadmium)
- [ ] Herbicides
- [ ] Marijuana
- [ ] Medications (such as narcotics for pain and benzodiazepines for anxiety or insomnia)
- [ ] Mold
- [ ] Paint and solvent fumes
- [ ] Pesticides
- [ ] Pesticide and herbicide residues in farms and backyards
- [ ] Silicone breast implants that have leaked
- [ ] Tainted water
- [ ] Vehicle exhaust
- [ ] Welding or soldering fumes

KEY TOXIN TESTS

The organs that detoxify your body—especially the liver, kidneys, and skin—need to be supported to do their job. The tests below will tell you how these organs are coping with your body's toxic load.

LIVER FUNCTION

ALT (SGPT): Normal range: 7 to 56 units per liter (U/L)
AST (SGOT): Normal range: 5 to 40 U/L
Bilirubin: Normal range: 0.2 to 1.2 mg/dL
Zinc: Normal range: 60 to 110 mcg/dL (low zinc will limit detoxification in the liver)

KIDNEY FUNCTION

BUN: Normal range: 7 to 20 mg/dL

Creatinine: Normal range: 0.5 to 1.2 mg/dL

SKIN

Check for rashes, acne, and rosacea

TESTING FOR MOLD

Real Time Labs mycotoxin test: realtimelab.com for mold tests of human and environmental samples

TGF beta-1: Normal level: below 2,380; 0 is optimal. Mold exposure can raise this to more than 15,000

RISK FACTOR: MENTAL HEALTH

The health of your mind is an essential factor in the health of your brain and memory. Mental health issues, including but not limited to, depression, bipolar disorder, attention deficit disorder/attention deficit hyperactivity disorder (ADD/ADHD), early childhood trauma, posttraumatic stress disorder (PTSD), anxiety, and chronic stress can contribute to a higher risk of memory, cardiovascular, and other health problems. This is why you need to make sure your mind is as fit as it can be.

YOUR PERSONAL RISK CHECKLIST:

Which Mental Health Risk Factors Do You Have?

It is important to screen for mental health disorders, not only so you can get treatment to help with symptoms, but also to protect your brain and memory. One reason: When elderly people have depression, they may also show signs of cognitive impairment that can be misdiagnosed as dementia.

- [ ] ADHD
- [ ] Anxiety
- [ ] Bipolar disorder
- [ ] Childhood trauma
- [ ] Chronic stress
- [ ] Depression
- [ ] PTSD

RISK FACTOR: IMMUNITY/INFECTIONS

This risk factor is all about your body's defender, the immune system, which is always on the lookout for external invaders and internal troublemakers. When your immunity isn't what it should be, you may be more vulnerable to allergies, autoimmune disorders, and infections, and the last two can increase your risk for brain fog and memory issues. As mentioned earlier, 80% of people who have had COVID-19 later complain of memory and focus issues.

YOUR PERSONAL RISK CHECKLIST:

Which Immunity and Infection Risk Factors Do You Have?

There are five types of immune system breakdowns, including immune deficiency disorders like HIV, allergies (to things like pet dander and peanuts), immune system cancers like lymphomas and leukemia, autoimmune disorders, and infectious diseases. The latter two, if left untreated, can cause serious memory problems and dementia.

- [ ] Autoimmune disorders such as multiple sclerosis, rheumatoid arthritis, systemic lupus erythematosus, Crohn's disease, psoriasis, Hashimoto's thyroiditis, and type 1 diabetes

- [ ] Infectious diseases, including COVID-19, Lyme disease (and other tick-borne illnesses), toxoplasmosis, syphilis, Helicobacter pylori (H. pylori), HIV/AIDS, and herpes

KEY TESTS OF IMMUNITY/INFECTIOUS DISEASE

- [ ] Complete blood count with differential
- [ ] Erythrocyte sedimentation rate (ESR)
- [ ] Antinuclear antibodies (ANA)
- [ ] Rheumatoid factor (Rh)
- [ ] Vitamin D: A normal level is 30 to 100 ng/mL; an optimal level is 50 to 100 ng/mL

Screening for common infections: If your memory is not what it once was and you don't have the benefit of a SPECT scan, consider getting screened for infectious diseases that commonly affect memory, such as:

- Borrelia burgdorferi (the bacterium that causes Lyme disease)

- Chlamydophila pneumoniae

- COVID-19

- Cytomegalovirus

- Epstein-Barr virus

- H. pylori

- Herpes simplex 1 and 2

- HIV/AIDS

- Syphilis

- Toxoplasma gondii

RISK FACTOR: NEUROHORMONE ISSUES

Hormones are messengers—chemicals that are made by different parts of the body and sent to other areas to control your body's basic functions. The brain plays a significant role, both in sending out signals to release hormones and in being influenced by hormones from other areas of the body. Hormones work together in a delicate balance that can be upset if too much or too little of one or more is produced. When this happens, you may experience symptoms that affect how you feel, think or act, and you may be more prone to depression, Alzheimer's disease, diabetes, and other illnesses.

YOUR PERSONAL RISK CHECKLIST:

Which Neurohormone Risk Factors Do You Have?

There are many hormones that influence your brain, but these six are the most important: thyroid, cortisol, DHEA, estrogen, progesterone, and testosterone. Here are some of the risk factors you could have. You may not know you have one or more of them without getting bloodwork:

- ☐ Elevated cortisol and Low DHEA-S (adrenal fatigue)
- ☐ Excess estrogen
- ☐ Low estrogen
- ☐ Low progesterone
- ☐ Excess testosterone

- ☐ Low testosterone
- ☐ Overactive thyroid
- ☐ Underactive thyroid
- ☐ Perimenopause
- ☐ Menopause

KEY NEUROHORMONE TESTS

- [ ] Cortisol

- [ ] DHEA-S (note that normal blood levels can differ by age and sex)

- [ ] Estrogen and progesterone (women only)

- [ ] Ferritin level

- [ ] Free and total serum testosterone (men and women)

- [ ] Liver function tests

- [ ] Thyroid panel (includes thyroid stimulating hormone (TSH), Free T3, Free T4, and thyroid antibodies)

Quick Memory Tip:

Getting a baseline screening around age 35—and then reassessed every couple of years—can provide valuable information to help offset some of the symptoms that women often begin experiencing with perimenopause.

RISK FACTOR: DIABESITY

The word "diabesity" is a combination of diabetes and obesity, which are independent risk factors for failing memory and some forms of dementia. Diabetes damages blood vessels and eventually wreaks havoc throughout the body and brain, which can lead to Alzheimer's disease and vascular dementia, stroke, hypertension, and more. And being overweight or obese in midlife is associated with memory problems and dementia later on. Obesity can contribute to the risk of diabetes, too. The connection is so strong that some researchers are calling Alzheimer's disease "Type 3 diabetes."

YOUR PERSONAL RISK CHECKLIST:

Which Diabesity Risk Factors Do You Have?

- [ ] Aging
- [ ] Alcohol abuse
- [ ] Excessive consumption of sugar and high-glycemic foods
- [ ] Exposure to toxins
- [ ] Family history of diabetes
- [ ] Obesity
- [ ] Metabolic syndrome
- [ ] Sedentary lifestyle

KEY DIABESITY TESTS

☐ Body mass index (BMI): optimal = 18.5 to 24.9; overweight = 25 to 30; obese is over 30

☐ Waist to height ratio (WHtR): calculate by dividing your waist size (in inches) by height (in inches); a healthy WHtR is 0.5 or less

☐ Fasting blood sugar

- Normal: 70-105 mg/dL
- Optimal: 70-89 mg/dL
- Prediabetes: 105-125 mg/dL
- Diabetes: 126 mg/dL or higher

☐ Fasting Insulin

- Normal: 2.6-25
- Optimal: Less than 10

☐ Hemoglobin A1c (HBA1c)

- Normal: 4-5.6 percent
- Optimal: Under 5.3 percent
- Prediabetes: 5.7-6.4 percent
- Diabetes: Over 6.4 percent

Quick Memory Tip:

Low-glycemic foods (i.e. many vegetables) are generally better for you because they don't spike your blood sugar. Check out the glycemic index (GI), which rates carbohydrate foods on a scale from 0 to 100+ according to the way they affect your blood sugar. Try to avoid the carbs with a GI rating greater than 60.

RISK FACTOR: SLEEP ISSUES

Your brain needs sleep to stay healthy. Research shows that during your slumbers your brain washes away waste and toxins that have accumulated throughout the day. Chronic sleeplessness or insomnia raises your risk of everything from stroke to anxiety to cancer. Plus, sleeping less than seven hours a night has been associated with a higher risk of dementia.

YOUR PERSONAL RISK CHECKLIST:

Which Sleep Risk Factors Do You Have?

☐ Depression

☐ Hormonal imbalances

☐ Insomnia

☐ Poor sleep hygiene

☐ Shift work

☐ Sleep apnea

KEY SLEEP TESTS

☐ Get evaluated for sleep apnea if you snore loudly, stop breathing at night, or are chronically tired in the daytime.

☐ Assess the number of hours of sleep you need.

Even if you have risk factors for memory problems, with daily practice and intention you can make your brain stronger and healthier now—and more resilient to problems in the future.

Step 3 details some overall healthy lifestyle habits that Dr. Amen frequently recommends to his own patients, and that everyone can benefit from in their quest for a better brain and a better memory.

Dr. Amen's 7 Favorite Foods to Improve Memory

1. Blueberries They are loaded with antioxidants to fend against free radicals and aging, and flavonoids and polyphenols that protect brain cells, improve concentration, boost blood flow to the brain, and help to prevent memory loss.

2. Colorful vegetables, especially leafy greens, and brassicas such as broccoli, kale, cauliflower, red cabbage, and Brussel sprouts. Brassicas have been found to help your liver, and a healthy liver is associated with a healthy brain.

3. Low mercury fatty fish, like wild salmon, trout, and scallops, but be careful about where it is sourced and check on the potential mercury content by visiting the website, www.seafoodwatch.org.

4. Healthy oils, like olive, avocado, and coconut oil, which can help boost your memory and your mood. Avoid pro-inflammatory oils, such as corn, soy, and vegetable oil.

5. Nuts and seeds, especially walnuts. A quarter cup contains 2.5 grams of essential fatty acids. And pumpkin seeds been found to boost dopamine and help you focus.

6. Green tea. It is loaded with the natural antioxidants like polyphenols and catechins, contains theanine, which can help you focus (important for encoding memories) and relax.

7. Healthy chocolate (not processed). Raw cacao has been found to boost your memory, increase blood flow to the brain, improve stem cell production, and reduce stress. Try Dr. Amen's easy Brain-Healthy Hot Chocolate recipe:
   - Heat unsweetened almond milk on the stove.
   - Stir in a heaping teaspoon of organic raw cacao.
   - Add a few drops of stevia.
   - Enjoy guilt-free because it's only about 60 calories!

Dr. Amen's 7 Favorite Supplements to Support Memory

Decades of clinical research have found that these 7 supplements can support—and enhance—your memory. Here are the ones Dr. Amen takes every day:

1. Saffron: Not only can it help with mood and memory, but some studies have also found it can help sexual performance.

2. Omega-3 fatty acids: Hundreds of studies have found that it helps support memory, mood, eyes, and heart, as well as your hair, skin, and nails.

3. B vitamins, especially B6, B12, and folate: In the proper dosages, they've been found to decrease the progression of mild memory problems to more serious ones, such as mild cognitive impairment to Alzheimer's disease.

4. Ginkgo biloba: Research with brain SPECT imaging showed ginkgo increases blood flow to the brain, which is critical for a healthy memory.

5. Choline: This is an essential nutrient that converts into acetylcholine, a neurotransmitter that is critical for memory and learning.

6. Probiotics. There is an important connection between the health of your gut, and your brain health.

7. Smart mushrooms: Specifically, reishi, cordyceps, and especially lion's mane mushrooms have been found to support memory, focus, and blood flow.

Dr. Amen's Most Recommended Exercise Strategies for a Healthier Brain and Body

Everyone can benefit from at least 30 minutes of daily exercise. The following types support not only your body, but also are excellent way to strengthen your brain and memory too!

Burst or Interval Training: 30- to 60-second bursts at go-for-broke intensity followed by a few minutes of lower-intensity exertion. For example, during a 30- or 40-minute walk, take four or five one-minute periods to "burst" (walking or running as fast as you can), and walk at a normal pace between bursts.

Coordination Exercises: dancing, table tennis (ping-pong), pickleball, and tennis

Mindful Exercises: Yoga and Tai Chi

Strength Training: Two 30- or 45-minute weight-lifting sessions a week, a day or two apart—one for your upper body—arms, upper back, and chest—and the other day for your lower body—legs, abdominals, and lower back.

STEP 4
MEMORY MAKEOVER TIPS FOR BRIGHT MINDS RISK FACTORS

Step 4 provides specific memory makeover tips for each of the BRIGHT MINDS risk factors that can be incorporated into your daily life. As you read through this section, pay careful attention to the specific makeover tips that are geared to reduce your personal BRIGHT MINDS risk factors.

MEMORY MAKEOVER TIPS FOR BLOOD FLOW

- Get treatment and start prevention strategies early to minimize the risk of heart disease, atrial fibrillation, high cholesterol, prehypertension or hypertension, and erectile dysfunction.

- if you are overweight—a BMI of 25 or higher—it's important to lose the extra weight.

- Eat a nutrient-rich diet that keeps inflammation in check.

- Improve sleep hygiene to get 7-8 hours of sleep every night.

- Meditate or pray for 10-20 minutes daily.

- Avoid or eliminate alcohol, caffeine, fruit juices, and sodas, including diet sodas.

- Drink plenty of water.

- Avoid or eliminate baked goods, fast foods, fried foods, and trans fats.

- Limit salt intake to 1,500-2,300 mg. a day.

- Eat more plant-based foods for their fiber and healthy nutrients, which improve blood flow.

- Consider blood pressure-lowering supplements, such as magnesium, potassium, CoQ10, vitamins C and D, and aged garlic.

- If you have had any events during which you had a loss of oxygen or have sleep apnea consider doing hyperbaric oxygen treatment. And, if you have sleep apnea it is important to use a CPAP device when you sleep.

- Exercise regularly each week for at least 30 minutes at a time (see below).

Take Advantage of the Blood Flow Benefits of Exercise

Here are just a few of the ways in which exercise can help your blood vessels and your brain. It can:

- improve blood pressure

- improve the heart's ability to pump blood throughout the body and brain, which boosts oxygen and nutrient delivery

- increase the flexibility of blood vessels, which lowers the risk for high blood pressure, stroke, and heart disease

- stimulate the brain's ability to grow new brain cells (neurons)

- help improve mood, focus, and cognitive flexibility

Quick Memory Tip:

Getting a baseline screening around age 35—and then reassessed every couple of years—can provide valuable information to help offset some of the symptoms that women often begin experiencing with perimenopause.

Consider Taking Nutraceuticals that Improve Blood Flow

- Cocoa flavanols: 1oz. of sugar-free, dairy-free dark chocolate every day

- Ginkgo biloba extract: 60 to 120 mg twice a day

- Green tea catechins (GTC): Up to 600 mg a day

- Omega-3 fatty acids: 1,400 to 2,800 mg a day in roughly a 60/40 EPA:DHA ratio

- Probiotics: 3 billion live organisms a day, with both Lactobacillus and Bifidobacterium bacterial strains

- Resveratrol: 75 mg a day

Add More of These Heart-Healthy Foods and Spices to Your Diet

- **Arginine-rich foods:** beets (and beet juice), pork, turkey, chicken, beef, salmon, halibut, trout, steel-cut oats, clams, watermelon, pistachios, walnuts, seeds, kale, spinach, celery, cabbage, and radishes

- **Fiber-rich foods:** psyllium husk, navy beans, raspberries, broccoli, spinach, lentils, green peas, pears, winter squash, cabbage, green beans, avocados, coconut, figs, artichokes, chickpeas, and hemp and chia seeds

- **Garlic**

- **Maca:** a root vegetable native to Peru, usually available in powder form

- **Magnesium-rich foods:** pumpkin and sunflower seeds, almonds, spinach, Swiss chard, sesame seeds, beet greens, summer squash, quinoa, black beans, and cashews

- **Omega-3–rich foods:** flaxseeds, walnuts, salmon, sardines, beef, shrimp, walnut oil, chia seeds, and avocado oil

- **Polyphenol-rich foods:** blueberries, green tea, coffee, curcumin, and thyme

- **Potassium-rich foods:** beet greens, Swiss chard, spinach, bok choy, beets, Brussels sprouts, broccoli, celery, cantaloupe, tomatoes, salmon, banana, onions, green peas, sweet potato, avocados, and lentils

- **Spices:** cayenne pepper, ginger, garlic, turmeric, coriander and cardamom, cinnamon, rosemary, and bergamot

- **Vitamin B6, B12, and folate-rich foods:** leafy greens, cabbage, bok choy, bell peppers, cauliflower, lentils, asparagus, garbanzo beans, spinach, broccoli, parsley, cauliflower, salmon, sardines, lamb, tuna, beef, and eggs

- **Vitamin C–rich foods:** natural blood thinners to boost circulation, including oranges, tangerines, kiwifruit, berries, red and yellow bell peppers, broccoli, tomatoes, peas, and dark green leafy vegetables, such as spinach and kale

- **Vitamin E–rich foods:** green leafy vegetables, almonds, hazelnuts, and sunflower seeds

MEMORY MAKEOVER TIPS FOR RETIREMENT/AGING

To combat risks from retirement, social isolation, or loneliness:

- Be physically active.
- Develop new friendships.
- Get involved with your family, community, church, or other groups.
- Take a class to engage in new learning and meet new people.
- Volunteer to help others in your community.

If your iron level is too high:

- Avoid foods with naturally high levels of iron: red meat, spinach, chard, cumin, lentils, chickpeas, broccoli, soybeans, collard greens, leeks, beans, sprouts, asparagus, kelp, pumpkin and sesame seeds, and olives.

- Check the label of your multivitamin/mineral to see if it's high in iron. If it is, consider taking a different one.

- Consider donating blood.

- Limit the use of iron pans when cooking.

- Minimize alcohol consumption because it increases the absorption of iron from your diet.

- Read the labels of processed food products (like cereal) to see if they are "iron fortified" and avoid them if they are.

If your iron level is too low:

- Consider taking an iron supplement to increase it to a healthier level.

If testing revealed that your telomeres (casings at the ends of your chromosomes) are shrinking:

- Address your stress by learning and practicing stress reduction techniques, such as mindfulness meditation.

- Avoid exposure to heavy metals.

- Avoid alcohol, processed foods, sodas, and trans fats.

- Eat plenty of antioxidant-rich foods and spices (see recommended list below).

- Exercise regularly.

- Get 7 to 8 hours of sleep a night.

- If you smoke cigarettes, get support to help you quit ASAP.

- Lose weight If your BMI is 25 or higher.

- Take a multivitamin/mineral daily.

- Treat any infections promptly.

Consider Taking Nutraceuticals that Help Improve Your Memory and Brain Function

- Acetyl-L-carnitine (ALCAR): 500 to 2,000 mg a day

- Alpha GPC (alpha-glycerylphosphorylcholine): 600 mg once or twice a day

- Bacopa (bacopa monnieri): 250 to 500 mg per day of the standardized extract Synapsa

- Huperzine A: 50 to 100 mcg twice a day

- N-acetylcysteine (NAC): 600 to 1,800 mg a day; try starting at 600 mg twice a day

- Phosphatidylserine (PS): 200 to 300 mg a day

- Saffron: 30 mg a day of a concentrate produced from the flower or 176.5 mg a day of Satiereal (patented preparation)

- Sage: 300 to 600 mg of dried sage leaf in capsules, or 25 to 50 microliters; *if you have high blood pressure or a seizure disorder use only under a physician's supervision.*

Quick Memory Tip:

To help your brain rid itself of cellular toxins that accumulate during the day, try fasting for 12 to 16 hours between dinner and breakfast. For example, if you eat dinner at 7 p.m., plan to have breakfast sometime between 7 and 11 a.m.

Add More of These Anti-Aging Foods and Spices to Your Diet:

- **Allicin-rich foods**: raw, crushed garlic, onions, and shallots

- **Antioxidant-rich foods**: acai fruit, parsley, cocoa powder, raspberries, walnuts, blueberries, artichokes, cranberries, kidney beans, blackberries, pomegranates, chocolate, olive and hemp oils (don't use either for cooking at high temperatures), dandelion greens, and green tea

- **Antioxidant-rich spices:** cloves, oregano, rosemary, thyme, cinnamon, turmeric, sage, garlic, ginger, and fennel

- **Choline-rich foods:** (to support acetylcholine and memory) shrimp, eggs, scallops, chicken, turkey, beef, cod, salmon, shiitake mushrooms, chickpeas, lentils, and collard greens

- **Polyphenols-rich foods:** blueberries, green tea, coffee, curcumin, and thyme

- **Vitamin B6, B12, and folate-rich foods:** leafy greens, cabbage, bok choy, bell peppers, cauliflower, lentils, asparagus, garbanzo beans, spinach, broccoli, salmon, lamb, tuna, beef, sardines, and eggs

MEMORY MAKEOVER TIPS FOR INFLAMMATION

If you have leaky gut:

- Avoid things that hurt your gut, such as medications (e.g., antibiotics, NSAIDS, proton pump inhibitors), toxins, stress, intestinal infections, gluten, excessive alcohol—and more.

- Eat more prebiotic foods, such as beans, apples, onions, and root vegetables, which feed good probiotic bacteria.

- Increase the healthy bacteria in your gastrointestinal tract by taking a probiotic supplement or eating fermented foods with live bacteria, such as kefir, kombucha tea, pickled fruits/ veggies, and unsweetened yogurt.

- Take antibiotics only when indicated and necessary.

If your homocysteine level is elevated:

- Optimize your levels of B vitamins—especially B6, B12, and folate—to help lower homocysteine.

If you have low levels of omega-3 fatty acids EPA and DHA:

- Eat more cold-water fish, including salmon, tuna, mackerel, sardines, and herring. Check www.seafoodwatch.org to make sure the fish you plan to consume isn't contaminated with mercury or other toxins.

- Take an omega-3 fatty supplement: 1,400 to 2,800 mg a day in roughly a 60/40 EPA:DHA ratio.

If you have bleeding gums or periodontal (gum) disease:

- Brush your teeth twice a day and floss daily.

- See a dentist twice a year for regular checkups and cleanings.

Quick Memory Tip:

To help strengthen your memory and keep your brain sharp, try to have an Omega-3 Index of at least 8.

Consider Taking Nutraceuticals

- Curcumin: 500 to 2,000 mg a day of a highly bioavailable supplement such as Longvida

- Lower a high homocysteine level with folate (800 micrograms [mcg] a day of methyl folate), vitamin B12 (500 mcg a day of methyl cobalamin), and vitamin B6 (20 mg a day or pyridoxine hydrochloride or pyridoxal-5-phosphate)

- Omega-3 fatty acids: 1,400 to 2,800 mg a day in roughly a 60/40 EPA:DHA ratio

- Probiotics: 3 billion live organisms a day; look for both Lactobacillus and Bifidobacterium bacterial strains

Add More of These Inflammation-Fighting Foods and Spices to Your Diet

- **Allicin-rich foods:** raw, crushed garlic, onions, and shallots

- **Anti-inflammatory spices:** turmeric, cayenne, ginger, cloves, cinnamon, oregano, pumpkin pie spice, rosemary, sage, and fennel

- **Fiber-rich foods:** psyllium husk, navy beans, raspberries, broccoli, spinach, lentils, green peas, pears, winter squash, cabbage, green beans, avocados, coconut, figs, artichokes, chickpeas, and hemp and chia seeds

- **Folate-rich foods:** spinach, dark leafy greens, asparagus, turnips, beets, mustard greens, Brussels sprouts, lima beans, beef liver, root vegetables, kidney beans, white beans, salmon, and avocado

- **Magnesium-rich foods:** pumpkin and sunflower seeds, almonds, spinach, Swiss chard, sesame seeds, beet greens, summer squash, quinoa, black beans, and cashews

- **Omega-3-rich foods:** flaxseeds, walnuts, salmon, sardines, beef, shrimp, walnut oil, chia seeds, and avocado oil

- **Prebiotic-rich foods:** dandelion greens, asparagus, chia seeds, beans, cabbage, psyllium, artichokes, raw garlic, onions, leeks, and root vegetables, such as sweet potatoes, yams, squash, jicama, beets, carrots, turnips

- **Probiotic-rich foods:** brined vegetables (not vinegar), kimchi, sauerkraut, kefir, miso soup, pickles, spirulina, chlorella, blue-green algae, and kombucha tea

- **Tart cherry juice:** to lower levels of C-reactive protein (CRP)

MEMORY MAKEOVER TIPS FOR GENETICS

If you have a family history of memory problems, dementia, or you carry one or two APOE genes:

- Be serious about the health of your brain: Engage in sports or hobbies that call for new learning and protect your blood vessels.

- Exercise aerobically, do balance exercises, and strengthen your muscles.

- Get screened early (around age 40) with cognitive testing, questionnaires, and even SPECT imaging.

- Protect your head from injury and concussions.

Quick Memory Tip:

Carrying the APOE4 gene doesn't mean you will develop Alzheimer's—only about 25% of people who inherit the gene succumb to the disease. However, it is critical that you protect your blood vessels and take exceptional care of your brain.

Consider Taking Nutraceuticals Daily

- Blueberry extract
- Resveratrol
- Green tea catechins (GTC)
- Acetyl-L-carnitine (ALCAR)
- Curcumins
- Ashwagandha

- Ginseng
- N-acetylcysteine
- Coenzyme Q10 (CoQ10)
- Magnesium
- Vitamins B6 and B12
- Omega-3 fatty acid DHA

Quick Memory Tip:

Foods like processed cheese and microwave popcorn contain a flavoring called diacetyl that increases beta amyloid, a sticky brain substance linked to Alzheimer's disease.

Add More of These Brain-Boosting Foods and Spices to Your Diet

- **Foods to decrease beta amyloid:** salmon, blueberries, and curry

- **Magnesium-rich foods:** pumpkin and sunflower seeds, almonds, spinach, Swiss chard, sesame seeds, beet greens, summer squash, quinoa, black beans, and cashews

- **Polyphenol-rich foods and beverages:** cabbage, chocolate, blueberries, kale, onions, apples, cherries, coffee (no more than 2 cups/day), green tea, and red wine

- **Spices to help decrease beta amyloid:** sage, turmeric, cinnamon, cardamom, ginger, and saffron; cinnamon helps decrease tau aggregation

- **Vitamin B6, vitamin B12, and folate-rich foods:** leafy greens, cabbage, bok choy, bell peppers, cauliflower, lentils, asparagus, garbanzo beans, spinach, broccoli, salmon, lamb, tuna, beef, sardines, and eggs

- **Vitamin D-rich foods:** cod liver oil and portobello mushrooms

Also: *Consider trying a ketogenic diet, which is very low in carbohydrates. Animal studies have found it can decrease the accumulation of beta amyloid.*

MEMORY MAKEOVER TIPS FOR HEAD TRAUMA

To avoid injuring your head:

- Always wear your seat belt whenever you are in a car, truck, or other motor vehicle.

- Avoid climbing ladders or going up on a roof.

- Hold handrails when you go up or down stairs.

- Refrain from playing contact sports.

- Never text while walking or driving.

- Wear a helmet when you ski, snowboard, bike, etc.

If you have lost your sense of smell after a head injury:

- Help restore it by sniffing essential oils, including rose, cloves, lemon, and eucalyptus.

Quick Memory Tip:

After a head trauma like a concussion, spending time in a hyperbaric oxygen chamber where the air is up to twice the normal pressure might be helpful because it allows your body to absorb more healing oxygen.

Consider Taking Nutraceuticals

- A daily combination of ginkgo biloba extract, acetyl-L-carnitine, huperzine A, N-acetylcysteine, alpha-lipoic acid, and phosphatidylserine

- A daily high-dose multivitamin/mineral complex with higher levels of vitamins B6 and B12, folate, and vitamin D

- Omega-3 fatty acids: 1,400 to 2,800 mg a day in roughly a 60/40 EPA:DHA ratio

Add More of These Foods and Spices to Help Heal From Head Trauma

- **Choline-rich foods to boost acetylcholine:** shrimp, eggs, scallops, sardines, chicken, turkey, tuna, cod, beef, collard greens, and Brussels sprouts

- **Omega-3-rich foods to support nerve cell membranes:** flax seeds, walnuts, salmon, sardines, beef, shrimp, walnut oil, chia seeds, and avocado oil

- **Prebiotic-rich foods (they are anti-inflammatory):** dandelion greens, asparagus, chia seeds, beans, cabbage, psyllium, artichokes, raw garlic, onions, leeks, and root vegetables, such as sweet potatoes, yams, squash, jicama, beets, carrots, and turnips

- **Probiotic-rich foods (also anti-inflammatory):** brined vegetables (not vinegar), kimchi, sauerkraut, kefir, miso soup, pickles, spirulina, chlorella, blue-green algae, and kombucha tea

- **Spices and herbs to support brain healing:** turmeric and peppermint

- **Zinc-rich foods:** oysters, beef, lamb, spinach, shiitake and cremini mushrooms, asparagus, and sesame and pumpkin seeds

MEMORY MAKEOVER TIPS FOR TOXINS

To avoid ingesting or absorbing toxins:

- Buy and eat organic foods as much as possible.

- Drink 8 to 10 glasses of clean water daily.

- Eat more fiber: 21 grams a day for women and 30 grams daily for men.

- Get help for drug or alcohol abuse.

- Gradually replace amalgam dental fillings with ceramic ones.

- If you do not have an addiction to it, limit alcohol to two to four servings per week.

- Purchase food in glass, not plastic, containers.

- Read and understand food labels to avoid additives like BHA, BHT, MSG, red dye #40, and artificial sweeteners.

- Try a food detox for 2 weeks.

To limit your contact with toxins as much as possible:

- Avoid using products with volatile organic compounds (VOCs)—check labels on air fresheners, paints, cleaning products, and other potential sources of VOCs.

- Clean the air in your home: check for mold, change filters on heating/cooling units, and avoid having wood fires in the fireplace.

- Quit smoking—try hypnosis or nicotine patches.

- Replace aluminum and Teflon cookware—high heat may make Teflon release toxic fumes.

- Use fragrance-free natural household cleaners in your home.

Consider Taking Nutraceuticals To Support Your Vital Organs

To Support Your Liver:

- Artichoke extract

- Curcumin (in a bioavailable form like Longvida): 300 mg twice a day

- Folate (MTHF, methylfolate): 400 mcg a day

- N-acetylcysteine (NAC): 600 mg twice a day

- Selenium: 200 micrograms (mcg) a day

- Vitamin B12 (methyl cobalamin): 500 mcg a day

- Vitamin C: 1,000 mg twice a day

- Zinc: 20 to 30 mg a day

To Support Your Kidneys:

- Curcumin: 300 mg twice a day

- Fiber: seven grams (women) or ten grams (men) three times a day combined in food and supplements

- Ginkgo biloba extract: 60 mg twice a day

- Magnesium glycinate, citrate, or malate: 200 mg twice a day

- N-acetylcysteine (NAC): 600 mg twice a day

- Omega-3 fatty acids: 1,400 to 2,800 mg a day in roughly a 60/40 EPA:DHA ratio

To Support Your Skin:

- Alpha-lipoic acid: 300 to 600 mg a day

- Astaxanthin: 4 to 12 mg a day

- CoQ10: 100 mg a day

- Curcumin: 500 mg a day

- Epigallocatechin gallate (EGCG): 600 mg a day

- Grapeseed extract: 100 to 300 mg a day

- Omega-3 fatty acids: 1,400 to 2,800 mg a day in roughly a 60/40 EPA:DHA ratio

- Selenium: 150 micrograms (mcg) a day

- Vitamin D3: 2,000 IUs a day or more, depending on your level

- Vitamin E: 60 mg of mixed tocopherols a day

- Zinc: 25 mg a day

Quick Memory Tip:

Having a good sweat is one way your body clears out toxins, so it's important to exercise and take saunas regularly.

Eat More—Or Less—Of These Foods and Spices to Support Detoxification

For A Healthier Liver, Eat More:

- Berries
- Brassicas: any color cabbage, Brussels sprouts, cauliflower, broccoli, and kale for detox
- Caraway and dill seeds
- Green leafy vegetables (for folate)
- Protein-rich foods, including eggs
- Oranges and tangerines
- Sunflower and sesame seeds

For A Healthier Liver, Eat Less:

- Capsaicin (from red chili peppers)
- Conventionally-raised produce
- Dairy
- Farmed fish
- Grain-fed meats
- Grapefruit
- Processed meats

For Healthier Kidneys, Eat More:

- Blueberries, raspberries, strawberries, and blackberries
- Citrus fruits, except grapefruit
- Nuts and seeds: cashews, almonds, and pumpkin seeds for magnesium
- Sugar-free chocolate
- Garlic
- Ginger
- Green leafy vegetables
- Spices to support detoxification: clove, rosemary, and turmeric

For Healthier Kidneys, Drink More:

- Beet juice
- Water

For Healthier Kidneys, Eat Less:

- Excessive animal protein
- Excess phosphates found in processed cheeses, canned fish, processed meats, flavored water, sodas, nondairy creamers, and bottled coffee drinks and iced teas
- Too much salt

For Healthier Skin, Eat More:

- Almonds, walnuts, and sunflower seeds
- Colorful fruits and vegetables for antioxidants: especially organic berries, kiwifruit, oranges, tangerines, pomegranates, broccoli, and peppers
- Olive oil
- Sugar-free chocolate
- Wild salmon
- Avocados

For Healthier Skin, Drink More:

- Green tea
- Water

MEMORY MAKEOVER TIPS FOR MENTAL HEALTH

If You Have ADD/ADHD:

- Adopt brain-healthy habits.

- Exercise regularly.

- Find an ADD/ADHD coach to work with.

- Take medication if you need it.

- Try eating a higher-protein, lower-carbohydrate diet.

Consider Taking Nutraceuticals to Support Focus and Attention

- Iron (if ferritin levels are low)

- Magnesium

- Omega-3 fatty acids (higher in EPA than DHA)

- Phosphatidylserine

- Zinc

If You Have Depression:

- Adopt brain-healthy habits.

- Eat a diet that is rich in antioxidants and tomatoes.

- Do acupuncture treatments.

- Exercise regularly.

- Take medication, if you need it (if you do, be sure to take methylfolate too).

- Try cognitive behavioral therapy (CBT).

Consider Taking Nutraceuticals to Support Healthy Moods

- Magnesium

- Omega-3 fatty acids (higher in EPA than DHA), especially when inflammation markers, such as CRP, are high.

- Optimize vitamin D levels

- Saffron

- SAMe (s-adenosyl methionine), especially for males

If You Have Bipolar Disorder:

- Adopt brain-healthy habits.

- Consider taking omega-3 fatty acids EPA and DHA.

- Exercise regularly.

- Take medication if you need it

If You have PTSD or had Childhood Trauma:

- Adopt brain-healthy habits.

- Begin a meditation practice. One of Dr. Amen's favorites is a Kundalini meditation called Kirtan Kriya (see Day 227 in *Change Your Brain Every Day* to learn how to do it). Spending just 12-minutes a day doing this meditation can calm your emotional brain.

- Consider doing EMDR therapy (eye movement desensitization and reprocessing) to help you heal from the traumatic experience(s) you had. This therapy is offered by trained clinicians at Amen Clinics.

- Learn how to eliminate the automatic negative thoughts (ANTs) that steal your happiness *and* your memory. Whenever you feel sad, mad, nervous, or out of control, write down the ANT that is causing you distress and reality-test it by using the effective 5-Question strategy described on Day 117 in *Change Your Brain Every Day.*

- Take medication if you need it.

If You Have Anxiety or Chronic Stress:

- Adopt brain-healthy habits.

- Begin a prayer or mindfulness meditation practice.

- Drink green tea.

- Eat an ounce of healthy dark chocolate every day.

- Exercise regularly.

- Keep a journal to record your thoughts and feelings.

- Listen to soothing music.

- Turn off your mobile phone, tablet, and computer to reduce your daily screen time.

- Walk in nature.

- When you wake up, say to yourself: "Today is going to be a great day."

- Write down at least 3 things you feel grateful for every day.

Consider Taking Nutraceuticals for Anxiousness and Stress

- If you have a lot of anxiousness (a pervasive sense of tension and nervousness), consider supplements to boost GABA, such as GABA itself, magnesium, and theanine from green tea.

- If you worry a lot and have difficulty letting go of bothersome thoughts, consider supplements to boost serotonin, such as 5-hydroxytryptophan (5-HTP) or saffron.

- Optimize your DHEA-S level to the high-normal range.

Quick Memory Tip:
Having sex with your significant other can decrease stress hormones and might even boost your hippocampus—a critical memory structure in your brain.

Add More of These Foods and Spices to Your Diet to Help Mental Health Issues

- **Antioxidant-rich foods:** acai fruit, parsley, cocoa powder, raspberries, walnuts, blueberries, artichokes, cranberries, kidney beans, blackberries, pomegranates, chocolate, olive and hemp oil (don't use either oil for cooking at high temperatures), dandelion greens, and green tea

- **Choline-rich foods:** shrimp, eggs, scallops, chicken, turkey, beef, cod, salmon, shiitake mushrooms, chickpeas, lentils, and collard greens

- **Dopamine-rich foods for focus and motivation:** turmeric, theanine from green tea, lentils, fish, lamb, chicken, turkey, beef, eggs, nuts, seeds (pumpkin and sesame), high-protein veggies (such as broccoli and spinach), and protein powders

- **Fruits and vegetables for mood:** Eat up to eight servings a day

- **GABA-rich foods for anxiety:** broccoli, almonds, walnuts, lentils, bananas, beef liver, brown rice, halibut, gluten-free whole oats, oranges, rice bran, and spinach

- **Green tea**

- **Maca**: a root vegetable/medicinal plant (usually available in a powder form), native to Peru, that has been shown to reduce depression

- **Omega-3-rich foods:** flaxseeds, walnuts, salmon, sardines, beef, shrimp, walnut oil, chia seeds, and avocado oil

- **Magnesium-rich foods for anxiety:** pumpkin and sunflower seeds, almonds, spinach, Swiss chard, sesame seeds, beet greens, summer squash, quinoa, black beans, and cashews

- **Prebiotic-rich foods:** dandelion greens, asparagus, chia seeds, beans, cabbage, psyllium, artichokes, raw garlic, onions, leeks, and root vegetables, such as sweet potatoes, yams, squash, jicama, beets, carrots, and turnips

- **Probiotic-rich foods:** brined vegetables (not vinegar), kimchi, sauerkraut, kefir, miso soup, pickles, spirulina, chlorella, blue-green algae, and kombucha tea

- **Serotonin-rich foods for mood, sleep, pain, and craving control:** Eat dark chocolate and tryptophan-containing foods, such as eggs, turkey, seafood, chickpeas, nuts, and seeds (building blocks for serotonin) along with healthy carbohydrates like sweet potatoes and quinoa

- **Spices to support mental health:** saffron, turmeric (curcumin), saffron plus curcumin, peppermint (for attention problems), and cinnamon (for attention problems, ADHD, and irritability)

- **Vitamin B6, B12, and folate-rich foods:** leafy greens, cabbage, bok choy, bell peppers, cauliflower, lentils, asparagus, garbanzo beans, spinach, broccoli, parsley, cauliflower, salmon, sardines, lamb, tuna, beef, and eggs

- **Zinc-rich foods:** oysters, beef, lamb, spinach, shiitake and cremini mushrooms, asparagus, and sesame and pumpkin seeds

MEMORY MAKEOVER TIPS FOR IMMUNITY/INFECTIONS

If you have an infectious disease or autoimmune condition:

- Address any issues you may have with the health of your gut.

- Consider getting tested for heavy metals.

- Make sure your vitamin D levels are optimal.

- Manage your stress with meditation, laughter, and other helpful strategies.

- Try an elimination diet to see if food allergies are lowering your immunity. Avoid foods like corn, dairy, sugar, gluten soy, additives, preservatives, and artificial colors for a month then slowly add one back at a time to see how it affects you.

- Work with an integrative or functional medicine doctor who can properly diagnose and treat you.

Consider Taking Nutraceuticals to Support Immune Health

- Aged garlic

- Anthocyanins: fruit and vegetable extracts, blueberries, cranberries, and grape

- Echinacea

- Folate

- Melatonin

- Probiotics

- Selenium

- Smart mushrooms, such as lion's mane, shiitake, reishi, and cordyceps

- Vitamin A

- Vitamin C

- Vitamin D3

- Vitamin E

- Zinc

Add More of these Immunity-Boosting Foods and Spices to Your Diet

- **Allicin-rich foods:** raw, crushed garlic, onions, and shallots

- **Immunity-boosting spices:** cinnamon, garlic, turmeric, thyme, ginger, and coriander

- **Mushrooms:** shiitake, white button, portabella, morel, chanterelle, cordyceps, and reishi

- **Omega-3–rich foods:** flaxseeds, walnuts, salmon, sardines, beef, shrimp, walnut oil, chia seeds, and avocado oil

- **Prebiotic-rich foods:** dandelion greens, asparagus, chia seeds, beans, cabbage, psyllium, artichokes, raw garlic, onions, leeks, and root vegetables like sweet potatoes, yams, squash, jicama, beets, carrots, and turnips

- **Probiotic-rich foods:** brined vegetables (not vinegar), kimchi, sauerkraut, kefir, miso soup, pickles, spirulina, chlorella, blue-green algae, and kombucha tea

- **Quercetin-rich foods:** red onions, red cabbage, red apples, cherries, red grapes, cherry tomatoes, teas, lemons, celery, and cocoa

- **Selenium-rich foods:** nuts (especially Brazil nuts), seeds, fish, grass-fed meats, and mushrooms

- **Vitamin C–rich foods:** oranges, tangerines, kiwifruit, berries, red and yellow bell peppers, broccoli, tomatoes, peas, and dark green leafy vegetables, such as spinach and kale

- **Vitamin D–rich foods:** fatty fish, including salmon, sardines, tuna, eggs, beef liver, and cod liver oil

- **Zinc-rich foods:** oysters, beef, lamb, spinach, shiitake and cremini mushrooms, asparagus, and sesame and pumpkin seeds

MEMORY MAKEOVER TIPS FOR NEUROHORMONE ISSUES

If you have neurohormones that are too low or too high, it is critical to prioritize the optimization of them by eliminating the things that cause problems:

- Avoid processed food, excess sugar, wheat, and unhealthy fats.

- Limit alcohol to 2 to 4 servings a week.

- Lose weight if you are overweight or obese.

- Quit smoking cigarettes or vaping.

- Scale back your caffeine intake to 1 or 2 cups daily.

- Engage in beneficial lifestyle behaviors:

    - Eat a healthy diet.
    - Exercise aerobically and lift weights.
    - Get 7 to 8 hours of sleep every night.
    - Incorporate a stress-management program.

To reduce your exposure to endocrine disrupters, such as pesticides, phthalates, BPA, and parabens:

- Avoid buying and storing food in plastic containers – choose glass containers instead.

- Buy organic food whenever possible.

- Check the Environmental Working Group website (www.ewg.org) to learn which fruits and vegetables have the lowest and the highest pesticide levels.

- Limit or avoid conventionally-raised produce and dairy.

- When taking hormone supplements, opt for bio-identical ones because they have fewer side effects.

> ### Quick Memory Tip:
> *Eating licorice and soy and drinking spearmint tea can lower your testosterone levels, so stay away from these.*

Consider Taking Nutraceuticals to Support Healthy Neurohormones

- Calcium D-glucarate: 500 to 1,500 mg a day

- DHEA-S: 10 mg a day or more (if needed based on lab testing)

- Diindolylmethane (DIM): 75 to 300 mg a day

- L-tyrosine: 500 mg two to three times a day

- Omega-3 fatty acids: 1,400 to 2,800 mg a day in roughly a 60/40 EPA:DHA ratio

- Probiotics: 3 billion live organisms a day, with both Lactobacillus and Bifidobacterium bacterial strains

- Zinc: 20 to 30 mg a day

Add More of These Neurohormone-Balancing Foods and Spices to Your Diet

- **Eggs**

- **Estrogen-boosting foods:** soybeans, flaxseeds, sunflower seeds, beans, garlic, yams, foods rich in vitamins C and Bs, beets, parsley, anise seed, red clover, hops, and sage

- **Fiber-rich foods, including those that contain lignin:** green beans, peas, carrots, seeds, and Brazil nuts

- **Hormone-supporting spices:** garlic, sage, parsley, anise seed, red clover, and hops

- **Prebiotic-rich foods:** dandelion greens, asparagus, chia seeds, beans, cabbage, psyllium, artichokes, raw garlic, onions, leeks, and root vegetables like sweet potatoes, yams, squash, jicama, beets, carrots, and turnips

- **Probiotic-rich foods:** brined vegetables (not vinegar), kimchi, sauerkraut, kefir, miso soup, pickles, spirulina, chlorella, blue-green algae, and kombucha tea

- **Progesterone-boosting foods:** chasteberry, plus magnesium-rich foods, such as pumpkin and sunflower seeds, almonds, spinach, Swiss chard, sesame seeds, beet greens, summer squash, quinoa, black beans, and cashews

- **Testosterone-boosting foods:** pomegranates, olive oil, oysters, coconut, whey protein, garlic, and brassicas, including cabbage, broccoli, Brussels sprouts, and cauliflower

- **Thyroid-boosting (selenium-rich) foods:** seaweed and sea vegetables, brassicas, and maca

- **Zinc-rich foods to boost testosterone:** oysters, beef, lamb, spinach, shiitake and cremini mushrooms, asparagus, and sesame and pumpkin seeds

MEMORY MAKEOVER TIPS FOR DIABESITY

If you are overweight and/or have a family history of diabetes:

- Drink more water—and don't drink your calories.

- Exercise aerobically and lift weights.

- Limit your consumption of sugar and high-glycemic foods that turn to sugar, wheat and other grains, foods that are low in fiber, and processed foods.

- Lose weight slowly if you are overweight—aim for dropping one to two pounds each week.

- Take saunas to help detoxify your body.

- Talk with your doctor to find out if medication is necessary to manage diabetes.

Consider Taking Nutraceuticals to Support a Healthy Weight

- Alpha-lipoic acid (ALA): 300 to 600 mg a day

- Cinnamon: 1 to 6 g a day as a supplement

- Chromium picolinate: 200 to 1,000 micrograms (mcg) a day

- Epigallocatechin gallate (EGCG): 500 to 800 mg a day (only take the higher dose under a doctor's supervision)

- Magnesium: 50 to 400 mg a day

- Omega-3 fatty acids: 1,400 to 2,800 mg a day in roughly a 60/40 EPA:DHA ratio

- Vitamin C

- Vitamin D

Add More of These Diabesity-Fighting Foods and Spices to Your Diet

- **Fiber-rich foods to balance cholesterol and blood pressure:** psyllium husk, navy beans, raspberries, broccoli, spinach, lentils, green peas, pears, winter squash, cabbage, green beans, avocados, coconut, fresh figs, artichokes, chickpeas, hemp seeds, and chia seeds

- **Fruits:** apples, oranges, blueberries, raspberries, blackberries, and strawberries

- **Omega-3-rich foods:** flaxseeds, walnuts, salmon, sardines, beef, shrimp, walnut oil, chia seeds, and avocado oil

- **Magnesium-rich foods:** pumpkin and sunflower seeds, almonds, spinach, Swiss chard, sesame seeds, beet greens, summer squash, quinoa, black beans, and cashews

- **Polyphenol-rich food/drinks:** blueberries, green tea, and decaffeinated coffee.

- **Protein-rich foods:** eggs, meats, and fish

- **Spices:** cinnamon, turmeric, ginger, cumin, garlic, cayenne, oregano, marjoram, sage, and nutmeg

- **Vegetables:** best choices—celery, spinach, and brassicas (broccoli, Brussels sprouts, and cauliflower)

- **Vitamin D–rich foods:** fatty fish, including salmon sardines, and tuna, eggs, mushrooms (maitake, morel, and shiitake), beef liver, and cod liver oil

MEMORY MAKEOVER TIPS FOR SLEEP

If you have any of the following health problems that can interfere with sleep, discuss treatment options with your doctor:

- Anxiety, depression and other untreated or undertreated mental health issues
- Chronic pain
- Congestive heart failure
- Reflux and other gastrointestinal problems
- Restless leg syndrome
- Prostate problems
- Sleep apnea
- Thyroid conditions

Stop any lifestyle habits that cause chronic insomnia, including these:

- Avoid nicotine, chocolate, and alcohol in the evening.
- Don't eat a meal within two to three hours before bedtime.
- Eliminate caffeine after 2 p.m.
- Finish vigorous exercise at least four hours before you head for bed.
- Skip taking daytime naps because they can further disrupt your sleep/wake cycle.

Incorporate these 8 strategies to improve your sleep hygiene:

1. Avoid taking sleep medications like benzodiazepines—they can hurt your memory.

2. Establish a relaxing bedtime routine, such as by taking a warm bath or shower, sipping some warm almond milk, and turning down household lights low an hour before bedtime.

3. Go to bed at the same time each night and get up at the same time every morning.

4. Keep pets off the bed (and preferably out of the bedroom).

5. Make sure your bedroom is cool, dark, and quiet; use an eye mask, earplugs, or white noise device if needed.

6. Put away your gadgets (phone, tablets, digital watch) to block the screen light that can disrupt your sleep.

7. Try to resolve emotional issues before going to bed.

8. Use your bed for sleep and sex—and nothing else.

Consider Taking Nutraceuticals that Support Sleep

- 5-HTP (especially for worriers): 50–200 mg a day

- GABA: 250–1,000 mg a day

- Lemon balm (Melissa officinalis): 300–600 mg a day

- Magnesium: 50–400 mg a day

- Melatonin: 0.3–6 mg a day

- Vitamin D3: 3,500 IU a day

- Zinc: 20–40 mg a day

"My patients often like a combination of melatonin, magnesium, zinc, and GABA to help them sleep better." ~ Daniel Amen, MD

Add More of these Sleep-Boosting Foods and Spices to Your Diet

- **Chamomile or passion fruit tea**

- **Foods rich in melatonin (the hormone of sleep):** tart cherry juice concentrate (also improves antioxidant status), cherries, walnuts, ginger root, and asparagus

- **Healthy carbohydrates that increase tryptophan:** sweet potatoes, quinoa, and bananas

- **Magnesium-rich foods to reduce anxiety:** pumpkin and sunflower seeds, almonds, spinach, Swiss chard, sesame seeds, beet greens, summer squash, quinoa, black beans, and cashews

- **Serotonin-rich foods:** Combine tryptophan-containing foods, such as eggs, turkey, seafood, chickpeas, nuts, and seeds (building block for serotonin), with healthy carbohydrates (sweet potatoes and quinoa) to elicit a short-term insulin response that drives tryptophan into the brain. Dark chocolate also increases serotonin

- **Sleep-enhancing spice:** ginger root

STEP 5
CHART YOUR BRIGHT MINDS RISK FACTORS AND MAKEOVER TIPS

Finally! You are ready to start your personalized Memory Makeover program. For Step 5, begin by filling out the chart below using the information you have gathered regarding your personal BRIGHT MINDS risk factors. In the "My Risks" column, write in the aspects of each risk factor you have. In the "My Makeover Tips" column, write at least one makeover tip that you would be willing to try. Leave blank any risk factors that do not apply to you.

MY PERSONAL BRIGHT MINDS RISK FACTORS

Risk Factors	My Risks	My Makeover Tips
Blood Flow		
Retirement/Aging		
Inflammation		
Genetics		
Head Trauma		
Toxins		
Mental Health		
Immunity/Infections		
Neurohormone Issues		
Diabesity		
Sleep Issues		

TAKE ACTION

My Most Concerning Risk Factor(s) To Address Now

It isn't unusual to have more than one risk factor. And if you do, it may feel daunting to feel like you must tackle all of them at once. Rather than getting overwhelmed, consider starting with the one that is most concerning to you. Then as you progress on this 30-Day program and gain momentum, begin addressing each of the other risk factors you have. After 30 days, you'll be able to look back and see how far you have come by taking targeted steps to improve your brain, memory, and overall health.

Which risk factor will you address first?

_____

My Supplements/Nutraceuticals

In addition, to taking a 100% multivitamin/mineral complex that has extra vitamins B6 and B12, folate, and vitamin D, it's a good idea to take high-quality, targeted nutraceuticals that can have a positive impact on the brain. Check the list of nutraceuticals that are listed in each of the BRIGHT MINDS risk factors to see which ones are recommended for you.

Write down the supplements you will begin taking here:

_____   _____

_____   _____

_____   _____

_____   _____

_____   _____

_____   _____

_____   _____

My Brain-Healthy Foods/Drinks

In the memory makeover tips for each of the BRIGHT MINDS risk factors, there is a list of healthy foods and spices that are recommended to combat that particular risk factor. For each of your personal risks, select foods that you want to start incorporating into your diet now. Then keep adding more each week while avoiding memory-destroying foods like sugar, processed foods, hydrogenated oils, and other foods and beverages that cause inflammation in the body and brain.

Write down the brain-healthy foods you will incorporate into your diet here:

_____

_____

_____

_____

_____

_____

_____

After working this program for 30 days, re-take the cognitive tests you took in Step 1 and notice any changes in your scores. But don't stop there! Stay with the new habits you have acquired for your memory makeover and keep adding healthy lifestyle behaviors to your daily routine. In time, you will notice that your mind is sharper, your mood is better, and your energy has increased—all of which help you feel happier and more fulfilled in life.

MEMORY MAKEOVER RESOURCES

AMEN CLINICS

Memory problems, mental health issues, and cognitive decline can't wait. At Amen Clinics, we're here for you. We offer in-clinic brain scanning and appointments, as well as mental telehealth, clinical evaluations, and therapy for adults, teens, children, and couples. Find out more by speaking to a specialist today at 888-288-9834 or visit our website at amenclinics.com.

BRAINMD

Fuel your brain with high-quality, brain-directed nutraceuticals and other brain health products at BrainMD.com.